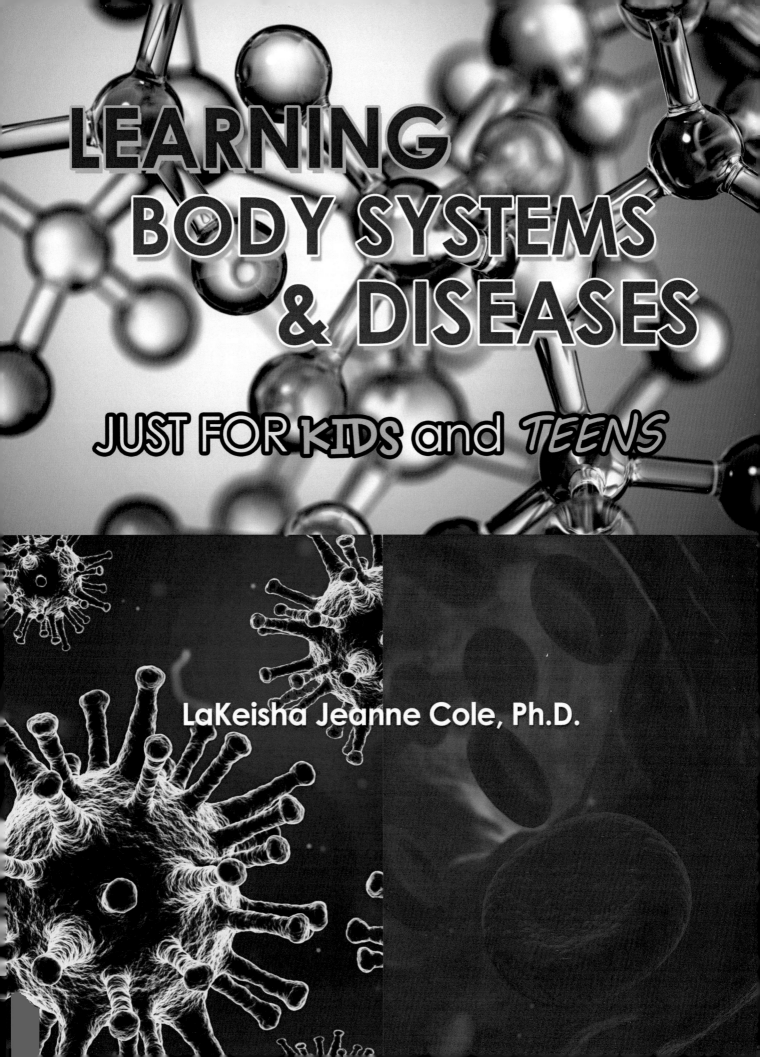

To order additional copies of this book, contact:
Xlibris
844-714-8691
www.Xlibris.com
Orders@Xlibris.com

Photograph on the back or last page of this book was taken by the author of this work, LaKeisha Cole.

ISBN: 978-1-6641-0857-8 (sc)
ISBN: 978-1-6641-0859-2 (hc)
ISBN: 978-1-6641-0858-5 (e)

Library of Congress Control Number: 2021919791

Print information available on the last page

Rev. date: 09/27/2021

This book is dedicated to my beautiful husband, William Clarence Cole III, and our sons, William Clarence Cole IV and Khalil Jontaé Cole, who continue to motivate and inspire me as a person to be all I can be. Thank you for being in my life and giving me what I needed and more than I could have ever hoped for in a family.

I LOVE YOU SO MUCH!

To all those who are learning about health and wellness, how the body is made and works, as well as the physical changes that can occur, and the individual continuous journey that goes along with it. Learn as much as you can, believe what you will, and NEVER stop believing and achieving your goals for better health and healing.

MAKE THE IMPOSSIBLE, POSSIBLE FOR YOU!

CONTENTS

Introduction

This book is written as basic information just for you. If you are a young child or teenager, it is designed to give you a simple and easy-to-understand reference to learn about body systems and diseases. This book is short and can be read over and over again. It offers pictures, highlighted words, and hints to say words to help you to say the words.

Learning about the body systems and disease will introduce you to how the body is made and how it works, and diseases to help you better understand them. There are many body systems, parts of the body, and diseases. Although all systems will be provided, only a few body parts and diseases will be discussed in this book. This is not an extensive list of *all* body parts and *every* disease in existence. Use this book as a guide for the preparation of basic human anatomy and physiology and disease subject matter.

If you are a young child, read this book with your parent(s) or trusted guardian. In learning about body systems and diseases, the subject of human life is discussed and must cover the female and male reproductive systems, their organs, and the diseases that affect the body parts related to those systems. Because puberty and adolescence can vary with stage and age group, this book is termed "for kids" (represented as "child") and that includes children under the age of 18 (for some, puberty can begin as early as age nine and late adolescence can range as high as 21 to 24 years). There is no limit to who can read this book, although it is specified for "kids and teens." Age group and grade level recommendations for this book range from nine years or fourth grade to 18 years (special circumstances may allow earlier or later age and grade). Human life and the reproductive systems, and disease, can be of interest for any age group and can affect individuals at any stage and age. This subject is for educational purposes only and should only be covered and shared with trusted persons.

Learning About Nutrition: Just for Kids is one of a series of children's books written by Dr. Cole. This book, Learning About Body Systems & Diseases: Just for Kids and Teens, can serve as a companion in helping to understand that book and vice versa.

ATOMS

Your body contains atoms. These units or elements make up your body at the most basic level. Carbon is one atom in your body. Hydrogen is another atom in your body. Oxygen is an atom in your body, too. There are many more atoms. Some of those atoms are calcium, magnesium, sodium, and potassium. See them on this periodic table on the next page.

Periodic Table

Legend:

- STABLE
- half life more than one trillion years
- half life in range of billion years
- half life in range of million years
- half life in range of thousands of years
- half life in range of years
- half life in range of days
- half life in range of hours
- half life in range of minutes
- half life in range of seconds
- half life in range of milliseconds
- half life undetermined

#	Symbol	Name
1	H	Hydrogen
2	He	Helium
3	Li	Lithium
4	Be	Beryllium
5	B	Boron
6	C	Carbon
7	N	Nitrogen
8	O	Oxygen
9	F	Fluorine
10	Ne	Neon
11	Na	Sodium
12	Mg	Magnesium
13	Al	Aluminium
14	Si	Silicon
15	P	Phosphorous
16	S	Sulfur
17	Cl	Chlorine
18	Ar	Argon
19	K	Potassium
20	Ca	Calcium
21	Sc	Scandium
22	Ti	Titanium
23	V	Vanadium
24	Cr	Chromium
25	Mn	Manganese
26	Fe	Iron
27	Co	Cobalt
28	Ni	Nickel
29	Cu	Copper
30	Zn	Zinc
31	Ga	Gallium
32	Ge	Germanium
33	As	Arsenic
34	Se	Selenium
35	Br	Bromine
36	Kr	Krypton
37	Rb	Rubidium
38	Sr	Strontium
39	Y	Yttrium
40	Zr	Zirconium
41	Nb	Niobium
42	Mo	Molybdenum
43	Tc	Technetium
44	Ru	Ruthenium
45	Rh	Rhodium
46	Pd	Palladium
47	Ag	Silver
48	Cd	Cadmium
49	In	Indium
50	Sn	Tin
51	Sb	Antimony
52	Te	Tellurium
53	I	Iodine
54	Xe	Xenon
55	Cs	Caesium
56	Ba	Barium
57	La	Lanthanum
58	Ce	Cerium
59	Pr	Praseodymium
60	Nd	Neodymium
61	Pm	Promethium
62	Sm	Samarium
63	Eu	Europium
64	Gd	Gadolinium
65	Tb	Terbium
66	Dy	Dysprosium
67	Ho	Holmium
68	Er	Erbium
69	Tm	Thulium
70	Yb	Ytterbium
71	Lu	Lutetium
72	Hf	Hafnium
73	Ta	Tantalum
74	W	Tungsten
75	Re	Rhenium
76	Os	Osmium
77	Ir	Iridium
78	Pt	Platinum
79	Au	Gold
80	Hg	Mercury
81	Tl	Thallium
82	Pb	Lead
83	Bi	Bismuth
84	Po	Polonium
85	At	Astatine
86	Rn	Radon
87	Fr	Francium
88	Ra	Radium
89	Ac	Actinium
90	Th	Thorium
91	Pa	Protactinium
92	U	Uranium
93	Np	Neptunium
94	Pu	Plutonium
95	Am	Americium
96	Cm	Curium
97	Bk	Berkelium
98	Cf	Californium
99	Es	Einsteinium
100	Fm	Fermium
101	Md	Mendelevium
102	No	Nobelium
103	Lr	Lawrencium
104	Rf	Rutherfordium
105	Db	Dubnium
106	Sg	Seaborgium
107	Bh	Bohrium
108	Hs	Hassium
109	Mt	Meitnerium
110	Ds	Darmstadtium
111	Rg	Roentgenium
112	Uub	Ununbium
113	Uut	Ununtrium
114	Uuq	Ununquadium
115	Uup	Ununpentium
116	Uuh	Ununhexium
117	Uus	Ununseptium
118	Uuo	Ununoctium

*HINT TO SAY WORDS:

Hydrogen (HI-DRO-gen)

Oxygen (ox-eh-gen)

Calcium (CAL-SEE-um)

Magnesium (MAG-nee-zee-um)

Potassium (po-TASS-CEE-um)

MOLECULES

These atoms join together to make new substances to help your body work well. For example, two hydrogen atoms can come together and join one oxygen atom to create water, also known chemically as H_2O. Your body is made up of 60 to 70% water. Every part of your body needs water to be healthy.

Did you know your body makes salt? The element sodium (Na^+) and chlorine (Cl^-) join together to form sodium chloride (NaCl), also known as salt.

*HINT TO SAY WORDS:

Molecule (ma-LEH-QULE)

Chlorine (klor-EEN)

Sodium (SO-dee-um)

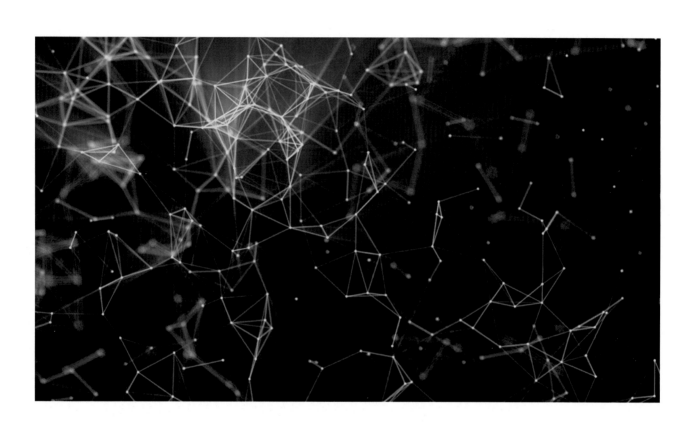

CELLS

When molecules of the body combine, they create the cell level. This important layer of the body contains its own materials that play major roles in the body, called organelles. Molecules in the cell nucleus (place of all cell activity) include genes, located on chromosomes, made of the gene code, deoxyribonucleic acid (DNA). Ribonucleic acid (RNA) carries instructions from DNA.

There are many organelles, and each is important to keep the body strong and work correctly for good health. One organelle is the mitochondrion, where the body makes energy for body activities. Other organelles include the plasma membrane, ribosomes, Golgi apparatus, lysosomes and endoplasmic reticulum. Some cells include blood, bone, fat, nerve, skin, and muscle.

*HINT TO SAY WORDS:

Deoxyribonucleic acid (D-ox-E-RI-BO-noo-CLEE-ic A-cid)

Ribonucleic acid (RY-BO-noo-CLEE-ic A-cid

Mitochondrion (MY-TOE-kon-dree-un)

Lysosome (LY-SO-SOhm)

Nucleus (new-CLEE-us)

Endoplasmic (en-doe-PLAS-MIK)

reticulum (reh-TIC-YOU-lum)

Golgi apparatus (GOL-gee) apparatus (a-puh-RAT-us)

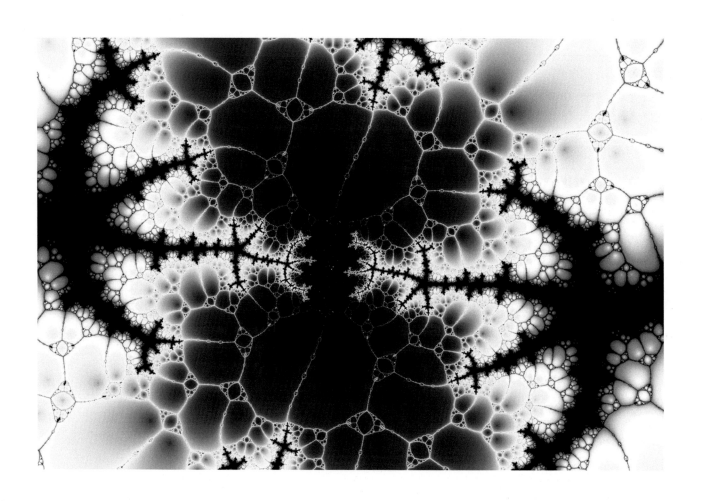

TISSUES

There are four types of tissue in the human body.

Epithelial – sheets of tissue that
cover and line inside parts

Connective – holds parts of the body together

Muscle – contracts (tightens) and relaxes (loosens)

Nervous – sends electrical signals through body

*HINT TO SAY WORD:

Epithelial (EP-i-thee-lee-al)

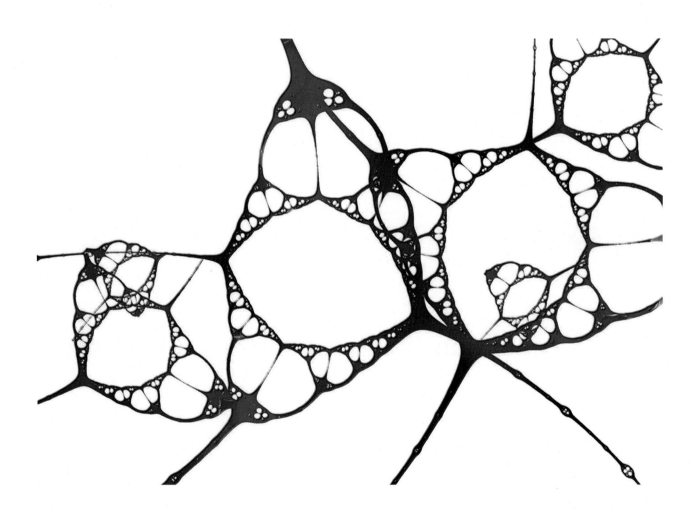

ORGANS

Tissues in the body work together to form and make organs. Every organ in your body is made of special tissues. These tissues create organs that have jobs in your body that allow it to work properly. Some of the organs in your body are your liver, kidneys, brain, and heart. Each organ has a special assignment and helps the body work together.

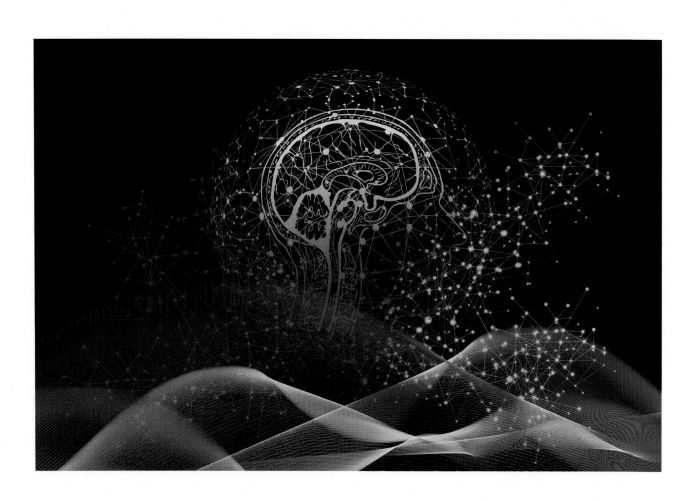

ORGAN SYSTEMS

All of the organs in the body belong to a special system. There are many systems in the body. Each has a unique job and must work with other systems that contain other organs to help the body work. For example, the pancreas is an organ the belongs to two different systems of the body. One system is the digestive system. The other system is the endocrine system.

You will learn about the other systems and organs as you keep reading this book!

*HINT TO SAY WORDS:

Pancreas (pan-kree-as)

Digestive (DIE-jes-tiv)

Endocrine (N-DOE-krin)

System (SIS-tem)

ORGANISM

All of the organ systems that are made up of organs, that are made of tissues, that are made of cells, that are made of molecules, formed by atoms, make up the complete organism, which is YOU!

You are an organism!

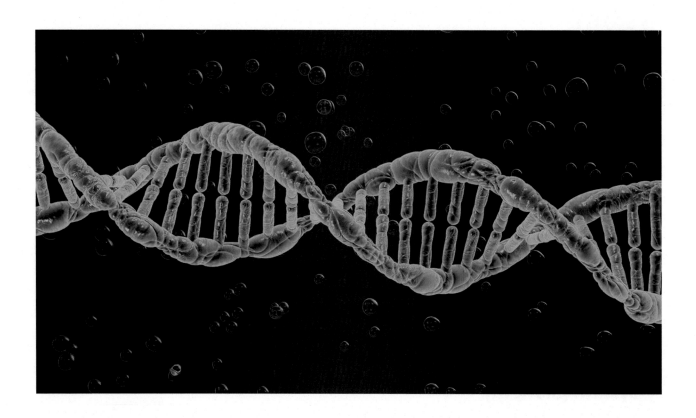

INTEGUMENTARY SYSTEM: HAIR, SKIN AND NAILS

This system is serves as a protective system. The body must be protected from materials outside that could cause harm. Parts of this system include hair, skin, nails, nerves, sweat and oil glands, rid the body of waste products and help keep body temperature stable.

Did you know the skin in the largest organ in the human body? The skin protects the organs and all parts of the internal body from the outside world.

Hair assists the body in keeping body temperature at normal levels. When things touch the skin, the hair acts as a sensor, or nervous system response that allows you to feel. Eyelashes help protect the eyes from harmful things that might enter to cause disease. Nose hairs filter particles from the air and trap them in mucus (thick, slippery fluid that protects and keeps moisture) so they can be removed from the nose.

Sebum is the oil released by the sebaceous gland and helps moisten the hair follicle (where cells divide and grow).

Nails are hard cells that grow and push to the surface and fill with the protein known as keratin.

*HINT TO SAY WORDS:

Sudoriferous (Soo-DOR-IF-er-us) glands = sweat glands

Sebaceous (See-base-shus) glands = oil glands

Nerves (NURVS)

Temperature (tem-pur-chur) or (tem-pur-choor)

Mucus (MYOO-cus)

Sebum (see-bum)

Follicle (fo-LIC-uhl)

Keratin (cayr-uh-tin)

SKELETAL SYSTEM

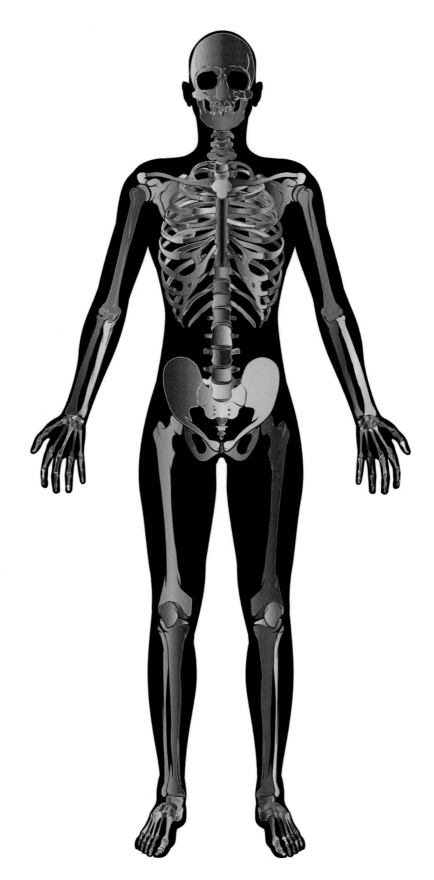

The skeletal system is the **framework** of the body. It consists of the bones that protect internal organs and hold the body together. Bone is a hard connective tissue, made of bone cells. These bone cells include osteoblasts (form bone), osteoclasts (break down bone), and osteocytes (mature bone).

The body contains places of **attachment** for the bones. These bones come together by **ligaments**. Ligaments attach bone to bone. **Joints** allow the bones to move. When you bend your arms and legs, rotate your neck and feet in a circular motion, your body must use different joints to allow this **movement**.

MUSCULAR SYSTEM

The muscular system is a system of contraction and relaxation. This system works with the nervous system to move all muscles. When a muscle in the body contracts, it will shorten and thicken as a nerve impulse is sent. Once this nerve impulse is removed, the muscle will return to its original length. This is known as muscle relaxation.

The organs in your body are made of muscle. Your body has three types of muscle. When your body breaks down food, it uses smooth muscle. This muscle moves without your motivation. It is involuntary. Another involuntary muscle is cardiac muscle, the muscle of the heart. Skeletal muscle is voluntary, attached to bone, and moves with your influence. A tendon attaches muscle to bone.

*HINT TO SAY WORDS:

Muscular (MUS-Q-LER)

Contraction (CON-TRAK-shun)

Relaxation (ree-LAX-AY-shun)

Involuntary (N-vol-UN-tayr-EE)

RESPIRATORY SYSTEM

This system is responsible for making sure that the cells of the body receive oxygen. Cells of the body require oxygen (O_2) for life activities to grow, reproduce, and maintain a stable environment (homeostasis). When the body uses this oxygen, it creates a waste product known as carbon dioxide (CO_2) that must be removed to maintain health. Oxygen is carried in the blood with other important substances to keep you healthy, and carbon dioxide is also transported in the blood in the opposite direction to be removed from the body. You inhale (breathe in) oxygen and exhale (breathe out) carbon dioxide though the lungs, tubes, and air sacs called alveoli.

*HINT TO SAY WORDS:

Homeostasis (home-e-o-STAY-sis)

Inhale (N-HAYL)

Exhale (X-HAYL)

Breathe (BREEth)

Alveoli (AL-VEE-O-LY)

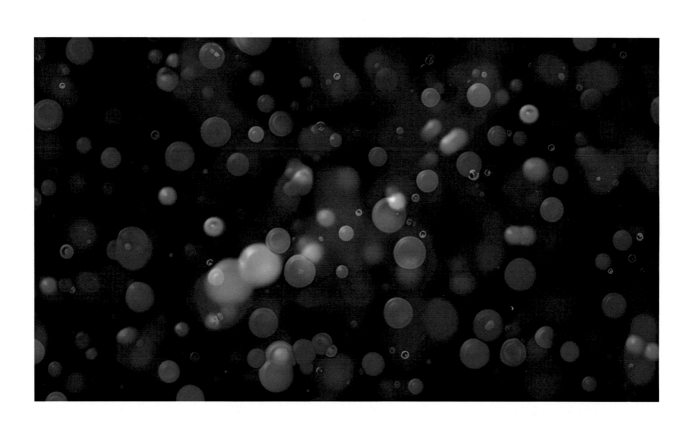

DIGESTIVE SYSTEM (GASTROINTESTINAL SYSTEM)

The digestive or gastrointestinal system is the system that receives food by mouth and breaks the food down with the teeth, passes it through the body, and uses the nutrients to provide the body with energy. Broken down food is formed into waste and removed from the body by the intestines.

Important organs of the digestive or gastrointestinal system include the pharynx, esophagus, stomach, pancreas, small intestine, large intestine, gallbladder, and liver. Each of these organs work with glands and chemicals to allow food to be processed by the body and used as fuel to support a healthy body. Salivary glands moisten food and enzymes break the food into smaller parts.

*HINT TO SAY WORDS:

Pharynx (fahr-eenks)

Esophagus (ee-soh-fuh-gus)

Stomach (stum-ik)

Pancreas (PAN-kree-is)

Small intestine (smawhl in-TESS-tin)

Gallbladder (gawhl BLAD-ur)

Liver (liv-UR)

Salivary glands (SAL-ih-VAYR-ee GLANds)

Enzymes (en-ZYMS)

URINARY SYSTEM

The urinary system is the system that filters the blood and makes urine.

There are a lot of activities that happen in the body to make this system work. The body must filter blood. To filter, the body will separate substances from the blood. Some of these substances are body fluids, wastes or toxic materials, salts and excess (too much) water.

The organs that work together to allow this to happen are two kidneys (filter blood and make urine), ureters (tubes leading to bladder), urinary bladder (holds urine), and the urethra (tubes that remove urine from the body).

*HINT TO SAY WORDS:

Kidney (KID-NEE)
Ureter (YOU-REE-TER)
Urethra (YOU-REE-THRA)

CARDIOVASCULAR SYSTEM

This system contains your heart and blood vessels. Arteries are tubes that carry blood to the heart and veins carry blood back to the heart. Your body pumps (pushes) blood through your body to make sure it carries all of the important things that your body needs to be healthy and strong. Every system must get these important things to give you energy when you eat food, help you breathe, and fight harmful things that can make you sick.

This transport system carries blood—which carries oxygen, carbon dioxide waste, blood cells, hormones, enzymes (proteins that break down fast), nutrients and other waste products through the body and removes harmful substances from the body.

*HINT TO SAY WORDS:

Cardiovascular (CAR-dee-O-VAS-Q-lar)

Heart (HART)

Artery (R-te-ree)

Vein (vayn)

Nutrients (NEW-tree-ents)

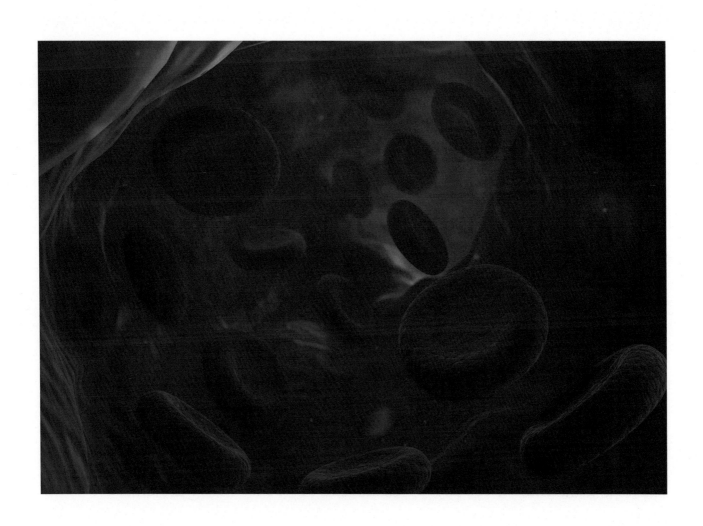

LYMPHATIC (IMMUNE) SYSTEM

The lymphatic system is the system created to help the body fight infection and disease. Immunity is the body's response to antigens (foreign harmful substances) that invade the body to make it sick.

Antibodies (immunoglobulins: IgG, IgA, IgM, IgE, IgD) protect the body against these antigens. Important organs and body fluids such as lymph and its white blood cells and disease-fighters, lymph nodes, lymphatic vessels that transport this fluid through the body, tonsils, spleen, and thymus gland help protect the body from harm.

Lymphatic system works like the game Pac-Man eating ghosts. White blood cells known as lymphocytes and macrophages DESTROY pathogens (disease-causing agents like viruses, bacteria, fungi, and parasites).

*HINT TO SAY WORDS:

Lymphatic (LIM-fat-ik)

Antigen (an-TY-jen)

Antibodies (AN-ty-BOD-eez)

Lymph (limFF)

Tonsils (tohn-SILS)

Spleen (spLEEN)

Thymus (thy-mus)

Lymphocytes (lim-FO-SYts)

Macrophages (mah-KRO-FAY-jess) or (mah-KRO-FAYJ)

Bacteria (bak-teer-ee-uh)

Viruses (VY-rus-iss)

Fungi (fun-GY)

Parasites (PAH-ruh-SYT)

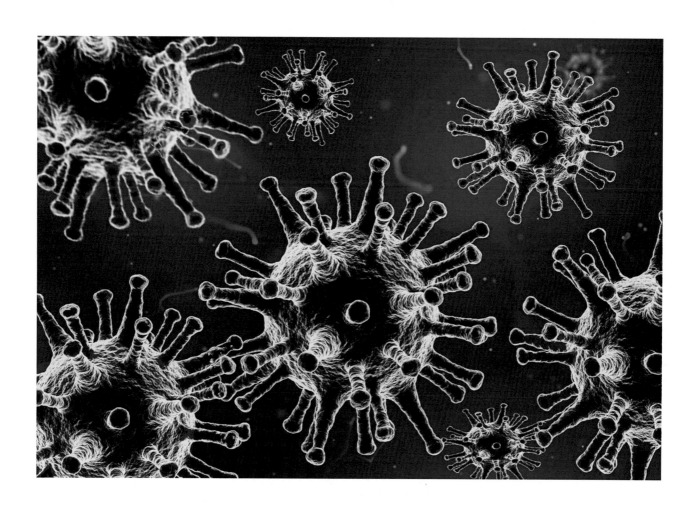

NERVOUS SYSTEM

The nervous system is the system that contains the central nervous system (brain and spinal cord) and the peripheral nervous system (everything outside of the brain and spinal cord). This system is responsible for sending and receiving messages (sensory) and interpreting and processing those messages (motor).

Every part of your body must receive a signal from the brain to do a certain job or perform a particular body activity. A hormone is a chemical messenger that tells the body what to do.

Neurons = nerve cells

Parts of a nerve cell include:

Axon, Dendrite, and Nucleus

*HINT TO SAY WORDS:

Neurons (new-rohns)

Axon (ax-ohn)

Dendrite (den-dryt)

Peripheral (pur-IFF-ur-ahl)

Nucleus (new-clee-us)

Sensory (sin-SOHR-ee)

Motor (MO-tohr)

Hormone (hor-mone)

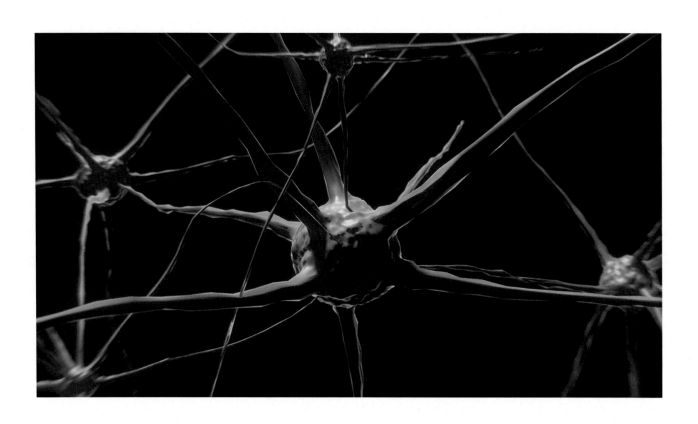

SPECIAL SENSES: SIGHT AND SOUND

The special senses include the members of the nervous system: sight (vision-the organs that allow you to see with your eyes), hearing (auditory-allow you to hear with your ears), smell (olfactory-allow you to smell with your nose), taste (gustation-allow you to taste with your tongue), and touch of the skin (fingers, toes) for sensation and vibration.

Senses have sensory receptors and other tissues with special neurons (nerve cells) that allow you to respond to your environment. This response is your stimulus. Nerve impulses allow you to become aware, interpret messages transmitted by the brain, and give the body balance.

Eye parts: cornea, lens, retina, and sclera

Ear parts: malleus, semicircular canals, cochlea, tympanic membrane and its cavity (space that holds it).

*HINTS TO SAY WORDS:

Vision (vih-zhun)

Auditory (awh-dih-TOR-ee)

Olfactory (OL-FAK-tor-ee)

Gustation (guh-STAY-shun)

Tongue (TUNG)

Sensation (sen-SAY-shun)

Vibration (vy-BRAY-shun)

Cornea (kor-NEE-uh)

Lens (lehNZ)

Retina (reh-tin-uh)

Sclera (SKLEER-uh)

Nerve impulse (NURV im-PULss)

Response (ree-spohnSS)

Stimulus (stim-YOO-lus)

Malleus (mah-LEE-us)

Semicircular canals (se-MY-sur-Q-lar CAN-als)

Cochlea (co-KLEE-uh)

Tympanic membrane (TIM-PAN-IK mem-BRAYN)

Cavity (CA-vih-tee)

ENDOCRINE SYSTEM

The endocrine system is the system that is responsible for glands (organs that make or release chemicals that send signals to and from the brain to do work in the body) and the tissues of these glands that make chemical messengers known as hormones in the blood.

There are many glands that help the body grow and develop, assist the body in using energy to fuel cells, delivery and spread of muscle and fat, sexual organs and their development, balance of fluid and ions (elements having a positive and negative charge), the body's inflammatory response and immune reaction. Glands of this system include pituitary, thyroid, parathyroid, adrenal, pancreas, and ovaries in females and testes in males.

*HINT TO SAY WORDS:

Chemical (kem-ih-cal)

Ions (eye-ohns)

Pituitary (pih-TOO-ih-TAYR-ee)

Thyroid (THY-royd)

Adrenal (ad-DREE-nuhl)

Ovaries (oh-vuh-reez)

Testes (tes-teez)

**Although puberty (adolescence) may begin as early as nine years of age, this subject matter is presented to aid in learning of body systems and diseases that affect these parts in various stages of the aging process.

REPRODUCTIVE SYSTEM

There is a female and male reproductive system. Each system is made of organs and other parts that participate in the process of creating human life. Before a baby comes into the world, it goes through stages in the mother's body that allow it to grow and develop. A fertilized ovum, diploid, haploid gametes, and embryo are *some* terms related to male and female reproduction.

The body parts of the female and male must come together to produce an embryo into a fetus (the beginning phase of life that will grow and develop until birth as a newborn baby).

Female body parts that help create and nourish human life include breasts, vagina, uterus, fallopian tubes and ovaries. Male body parts that help create human life include penis and testes in a scrotum (sac) that make sperm (joins an egg in the female reproductive tract to make new life).

*HINT TO SAY WORDS:

Female (fee-MAYL) or Male (MAYL)

Reproductive (ree-PRO-DUK-tiv) or reproduction (ree-PRO-DUC-shun)

Ovum (o-vum)

Fertilized (FUR-tuh-LYZD)

Diploid (DIH-ployd)

Haploid (HA-ployd)

Gametes (GAM-EETZ)

Embryo (ehm-BREE-O)

Fetus (fee-tuhs)

Breasts (BRESSts)

Vagina (vuh-JY-nuh)

Fallopian tubes (fuh-LO-pee-AN TOObs)

Penis (pee-niss)

Scrotum (scro-tum)

**Although puberty (adolescence) may begin as early as nine years of age, this subject matter is presented to aid in learning of body systems and diseases that affect these parts in various stages of the aging process.

DISEASES IN ALPHABETICAL ORDER

ATHEROSCLEROSIS
A-the-ro-scle-ro-sis

This form of cardiovascular disease affects the blood vessels in the human body. Remember, the vessels are the tubes that carry blood through the body. The arteries (tube carrying blood away from the heart) become filled with a plaque (fatty substance) and it blocks blood and form a clot (trapped red blood cells). When these vessels become narrow inside, they make it hard for blood to flow freely. This can make a person very sick because very important substances can no longer travel through the blood to be delivered to important body parts. This dangerous disease affects the cardiovascular system.

Signs and symptoms of this disease are chest pain, pain in the arms and legs or other parts of the body due to low blood circulation and oxygen, hard to breathe, tiredness, weak muscles, and confusion or dizziness.

*HINT TO SAY WORDS:

Atherosclerosis (AH-THER-O-skler-O-siss)

Vessels (veh-sehls)

Clot (CLOT)

Plaque (plak)

Circulation (sur-Q-LAY-shun)

BRONCHITIS
Bron-chi-tis

Bronchitis is a disease that causes inflammation of the bronchi. Inflammation is a response to the body, and it can be described as pain, swelling, redness, and heat. When the bronchial tubes that transport or carry oxygen of the lung tissues swell, this is what causes bronchitis. When the body is exposed to infections, some behaviors like smoking cigarettes, and allergies (body responds to a harmless antigen, or a harmless foreign substance in the body). The immune system is responsible for this kind of response. An example would be sneezing, watery and itchy eyes or skin, and runny nose.

*HINT TO SAY WORDS:

Bronchitis (bron KITE iss)

Bronchi (bron-KY)

Pain (PAYN)

Behaviors (bee-HAYV-yoors)

Cigarettes (SIG-R-ehts)

Allergies (al-UR-GEEZ)

Sneezing (SNEE-zing)

Itchy (it-chee)

CORONAVIRUS DISEASE (COVID-19)
Co-RO-NA-VI-rus

Coronavirus disease is a respiratory disease caused by SARS-CO-V2, a severe acute respiratory syndrome virus. The respiratory system is the system affected by this disease. The lymphatic (immune) system is the system that works to help fight the virus causing this novel (new) disease.

Signs and symptoms of this disease include coughing, fever, headache, sore throat, shortness of breath, chills and body aches, tiredness, loss of taste or smell, and other symptoms which may be different in people.

Experts recommend vaccination, wearing a mask, practicing social distancing of three to six feet, staying home for at least 14 days, and having two consecutive negative test results at least 24 hours apart.

*HINT TO SAY WORDS:

Respiratory (ress-PY-ruh-TOR-ee)

Immune (im-YOON)

Vaccination (VAC-SIN-ay-shun)

DIABETES MELLITUS
Di-a-be-tes Mell-i-tus

Diabetes mellitus is one of the leading causes of death affecting the endocrine and urinary system.

Diabetes Type I is also known as Insulin Dependent Diabetes Mellitus. Diabetes Type II is known as Insulin Independent Diabetes Mellitus, which is a preventable disease which can be managed with proper diet and exercise.

Diabetes is a health condition that results in high levels of glucose in the blood, resulting in high levels of insulin in the body due to little or no insulin production. Insulin (in-SUL-in) is a hormone made by the pancreas of the endocrine system, signaled by the brain when there is too much glucose (GLOO-KOS) (blood sugar) in the blood.

Signs and symptoms include excess urine, thirst, tingling hands and feet, fatigue (tiredness), slow healing of wounds, and weight loss.

*HINT TO SAY WORDS:

Diabetes (DIE-uh-bee-teez) mellitus (MEL-EYE-tus)
Diabetes (DIE-uh-bee-TIS) mellitus (MEL-uh-tus)

ENCEPHALITIS
En-ceph-a-li-tis

Encephalitis is an infectious disease of the nervous system and inflammation of the brain caused by West Nile Virus.

Most viruses are transmitted by insects like mosquitoes. Viruses travel through the bloodstream. Once in the body, the body will release disease-fighting organisms such as white blood cells to attack the virus that causes the disease. The body responds by inflammation, a reaction characterized by pain, swelling, heat, and redness.

Some symptoms include headache, fever, muscle and joint aches (AYks), confusion, and tiredness or feeling weak. As with most disease symptoms, people may experience different reactions.

*HINT TO SAY WORDS:

Encephalitis (EN-CEF-uh-light-us)

Mosquitoes (muh-SKEE-toes)

Confusion (cohn-FYOO-zhun)

FIBROMYALGIA
FI-BRO-MY-AL-gi-a

This health condition affects the muscular system. It can have a negative effect on the muscles and joints of the body, which will include the skeletal system. When these two systems combine, it is known as the musculoskeletal system.

The disease is characterized by signs and symptoms including muscle pain in different areas of the body such as the neck, back, or hips, and pain in joints and other soft tissues. Remember, tendons attach muscle to bone. Ligaments attach bone to bone. Both these tissue types can be affected by this condition. Sleep problems and difficult movement can be a burden due to pain and stiffness of body parts.

*HINT TO SAY WORDS:

Muscular (MUSS-Q-lar)
Muscles (muss-uhls)
Joints (JOYnts)
Ligaments (LIG-uh-ments)

GOUT

Gout is a type of arthritis, or inflammation of the joints. Gout is a metabolic disease that affects the body by a build-up of uric acid in the blood. This increase in uric acid forms crystals and can occur in the big toe. If these uric acid crystals move to the kidneys, they can create kidney stones. The musculoskeletal system is the system affected by this disease.

Signs and symptoms of this disorder include inflammation, which are pain, swelling, redness, and heat within the body.

*HINT TO SAY WORDS:

Arthritis (R-thry-tiss)

Metabolic (meh-tuh-BOL-ik)

Gout (GOWT)

Crystals (KRISS-tals)

Uric acid (YOO-rik AHS-id)

Musculoskeletal (muss-Q-lo-SKEL-eh-tal)

Metatarsal = bones of the foot of each toe that connect the ankle to the toe

Phalangeal (fu-lan-GEE-al) = phalanx (FAY-LAYnks) = one of the bones of the toe

Musculoskeletal (MUS-Q-lo-ske-le-tal)

HYPERLIPIDEMIA
Hy-per-lip-i-dem-i-a

Hyperlipidemia is a type of cardiovascular disease (remember, these are conditions affecting the heart and blood vessels) of the cardiovascular system.

This illness has high levels of lipids (fats) in the blood. Lipids in the body include cholesterol, phospholipids, and triglycerides which all travel in the blood. Cholesterol is used to make different types of hormones and is carried in the blood by proteins. High-density lipoproteins (HDL) is the good cholesterol and low-density lipoprotein (LDL) is the bad cholesterol.

Look at the periodic table and find phosphorus. Remember, atoms make up molecules, which combine to form cells. Cells are protected by the cell membrane (an organelle (or-GAN-ehl) also called the plasma membrane) made of phospholipids.

*HINT TO SAY WORDS:

Lipids (lih-pidz)

Blood (BLUHd)

Cholesterol (co-LESS-tayr-all)

Triglycerides (try-GLIS-ur-IDE)

Lipoprotein (lih-PO-PRO-teen)

Plasma (PLAZ-muh)

Membrane (mem-BRAYN)

Irritable Bowel Syndrome (IBS)
Irr-it-a-ble Bow-el Syn-drome

Irritable bowel syndrome is a disorder of the digestive or gastrointestinal system.

It affects the colon of the large intestine. When you eat food, it is broken down and must enter the blood where it can be delivered to cells for energy. As food moves through the tube of the digestive system, it reaches the intestines last. The food is combined with water, forms a liquid, then moves through the colon where it will get ready to exit the body.

Signs and symptoms of IBS include pain, bloating (full belly with gas), diarrhea (DY-uh-ree-uh) or watery stools, and constipation (hard to have a bowel movement or "poop"). Sometimes lactose (sugar in milk) products make it difficult to break down in the body, and stress, leading to IBS.

*HINT TO SAY WORDS:

Colon (co-LUN)
Intestine (in-TES-tin)

JAUNDICE
Jaun-dice

Jaundice is a health condition affecting the digestive system and has an effect on the Integumentary system.

This disorder appears to make the skin and the sclera (white part of the eye) turn yellow. The liver is the organ that plays a role in the color change. A substance known as bilirubin combines by liver enzymes (chemicals that break down) and is removed in bile (fluid made by the liver and stored in the gallbladder). When this bilirubin is not combined or joined, its levels rise in the blood. Too much bilirubin in the blood can be the result of damage to the liver and red blood cell destruction. The skin and the white part of the eye will become yellow in color.

*HINT TO SAY WORDS:

Jaundice (John-diss)
Bilirubin (Billy-Rubin like two names)
Liver (LIV-ur)
Bile (BYL)

KYPHOSIS
Ky-pho-sis

Kyphosis is a disease of the musculoskeletal system.

It results from the vertebrae (backbone) curve of the spine. From the back of the body, the bones that form the spine curve at the top. This health condition gives a humpback or hunchback shape to the back.

Signs and symptoms of this bone disease include back pain and difficult breathing may be a problem because of the pressure of bones that protect the lungs and other organs.

*HINT TO SAY WORDS:

Kyphosis (ky-FO-sis)

Vertebrae (ver-tuh-BREE) or (ver-tuh-BRAY)

KELOID is a mass of scar tissue that occurs when healing of a wound takes place affecting the integumentary system

After injury, the skin makes a scar as part of damage repair. An example of a traumatic event that occurs is ear piercing or a surgical cut. During this process, healing must occur, activating the inflammatory response. White blood cells go to the area to fight pathogens to prevent infection. When there is an overproduction of connective tissue (made of collagen fiber protein), a keloid may form, having a raised appearance.

*HINT TO SAY WORDS:

Keloid (KEE-loyd)
Collagen (kohl-uh-gen)

Leiomyoma (Fibroid tumor of uterus)
Lei-o-my-o-ma

Leiomyoma is a disease of the uterus of the female reproductive system. The smooth muscle tissue of the uterus affects the organ. There is an abnormal growth of cells that form a benign (non-cancerous) fibroid tumor.

Signs and symptoms can be different among women and depend on the size and area of the fibroid tumor, and how many may be present in the uterus. Pain, larger sized abdomen (waistline area), pressure in the pelvic, asymptomatic (no symptoms), and bleeding may be the result of these tumors. With time, they can shrink or disappear with age.

*HINT TO SAY WORDS:

Leiomyoma (LY-O-MY-o-muh)

Fibroid (FY-broyd),
asymptomatic
(A-SIMP-TOE-MAT-ic)

Benign (bee-9)

Uterus (yoo-TUR-us)

Abdomen (ab-DOH-men)

Pelvic (pel-vik)

Asymptomatic
(ay-sim-TOE-mat-ik)

Tumor (TOO-mur)

**Although puberty (adolescence) may begin as early as nine years of age, this subject matter is presented to aid in learning of body systems and diseases that affect these parts in various stages of the aging process.

MYOCARDITIS
My-o-car-di-tis

Myocarditis is a heart muscle disease of the cardiovascular system.

The heart muscle is made of different layers. The middle layer is the myocardium and it can become damaged. This damage can lead to inflammation of the heart muscle. The heart pumps blood using an electrical system with a rhythm (rih-thum). Once this disorder of the heart takes place, it can cause problems heart rhythm and the way the blood flows through the body. This disease is related to other diseases and infections, such as viruses.

Signs and symptoms of this condition are fever, fatigue, headache, difficult breathing, pain in the chest, swelling in the legs or arms because fluid builds up in the tissues, and abnormal heart rhythm.

*HINT TO SAY WORDS:

Myocarditis (MY-O-CAR-DIE-tiss)

Myocardium (MY-O-CAR-dee-um)

Inflammation (in-flam-ay-shun)

NAIL FUNGUS (*TINEA UNGUIUM*)
Tin-e-a Un-gui-um

Nail fungus, known as onychomycosis, or *tinea unguium* is a skin infection caused by fungus of the integumentary system.

Fungus is a pathogen that can affect the toenails. This fungus grows under the nail and can cause white patches and discoloration of the nail, turning brown, yellow, or green. The nail can become thick and crack.

It is important to take care of the nail to keep it from being completely ruined. This nail fungus can affect the other nails.

*HINT TO SAY WORDS:

Tinea unguium (tin-EE-a un-GWEE-um)

Onychomycosis (on-ih-KO-MY-KO-sis)

Fungus (FUN-gus)

Pathogen (PATH-O-jen)

OSTEOPOROSIS
Os-te-o-por-o-sis

Osteoporosis is a disease of the bone of the musculoskeletal system.

Pores or small openings in the bone cause it to break down and become thin. The bone loses important minerals like calcium and phosphorus, making it weak and more likely to result in a fracture (broken bone).

This disease affects older women and men. As women age, they have less of the hormone called estrogen that is important in the process of forming bone. This bone disease can cause the spine to bend and shortness in height.

Vitamin D is an important nutrient for strong bones and helps the body absorb calcium (just like a bath sponge absorbs or takes in water).

*HINT TO SAY WORDS:

Phosphorous (fos-for-us)

Estrogen (es-tro-gen)

PRESBYACUSIS
Pres-by-a-cu-sis

Presbyacusis is a disease of the ear that affects hearing. This health condition is a part of the special senses of sight and sound category.

With age, the ability to hear well can decrease. Sound can become less clear and eventually can be loss.

Presbyopia is a disease of the eye and affects vision or how well you can see. The lens of the eye becomes stiff and yellow and makes it hard to focus on objects with older age. This disorder should is NOT presbyacusis (ear).

*HINT TO SAY WORDS:

Presbyacusis (press-BEE-uh-Q-sis)

Presbyopia (press-BY-O-P-uh)

Vision (vih-zhun)

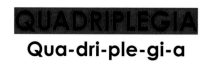
QUADRIPLEGIA
Qua-dri-ple-gi-a

Quadriplegia is a health condition of the nervous system that deals with injury to the spinal cord. This condition has its effect on the body beginning at the neck and ending with the extremities (arms and legs).

*HINT TO SAY WORD: QUADRIPLEGIA (KWAH-DRI-PLEE-G-UH)

QUARANTINE is an action taken when infected persons may have been exposed (been around something or someone) to a contagious disease and must be separated from others to determine if they are sick. Healthy people are kept away until risk (the thing or things that make the person more likely to get sick) for illness has passed.

*HINT TO SAY WORDS:

Injury (in-JUR-ee)

Spinal cord (SPY-nuhl KORD)

Extremities (x-TREM-eh-teez)

Quarantine (KWAR-N-teen)

RENAL DISEASE (KIDNEY DISEASE)
Re-nal Dis-ease

Renal disease is also known as end-stage kidney disease and kidney failure. The urinary system is affected by this disease.

The kidneys are the organs responsible for filtering the blood and separating substances to allow equal balance in the body. The system acts to rid the body of harmful wastes so they do not recirculate in the body's circulatory system. Just as you recycle trash, the kidneys work to make sure the pressure of the blood is good, toxins are removed by urine, red blood cells are formed, and pH of body fluids are balanced (not too much acid) from products made by the body. The body is smart. It keeps what it needs and gets rid of the rest. Extra materials are cleaned and reused to maintain health.

*HINT TO SAY WORDS:

Renal (ree-nuhl)
Urinary (Your-IN-AIR-ee)
Urine (YOUR-in)

SICKLE CELL ANEMIA
Sick-le Cell A-ne-mi-a

Sickle cell anemia is an inherited (gene from one or both parents) disease of the cardiovascular and lymphatic system.

Anemia is a condition that affects red blood cell ability to carry oxygen through the blood and deliver it to tissues. When red blood cells are made, they can become defective (not made perfect or correct in form). These flaws lead to problems in the blood vessels that carry the cells. Hemoglobin is a protein substance, that contains iron found in red blood cells, that binds oxygen. When red blood cells are not made well, improper shape can lead to too many cells, rupture and clot.

Signs and symptoms include pain, fatigue (fuh-TEEG), possible infections, and ischemia (is-KEEM-E-uh)— low blood supply to a body part).

*HINT TO SAY WORDS:

Inherited (in-HAIR-ih-ted)
Hemoglobin (HEE-MO-glow-bin)

TESTICULAR CANCER
Tes-tic-u-lar Can-cer

Testicular cancer is a disease that affects the male reproductive system and endocrine system.

The male produces the testes or testicles (egg-shaped glands found in the scrotum sac of the behind the penis). During puberty, this gland or sex organ makes sperm (the male reproductive cell or gamete) that will join the female gamete (egg cell) and create new human life.

Cancer is defined as the uncontrolled growth of abnormal cells in the body. Testicular cancer is cancer of one or both testicles. Signs and symptoms include swelling or enlargement of the area, tenderness, and a lump. There may or may not be pain.

*HINT TO SAY WORDS:

Testicular (tes-tic-u-lar)

Scrotum (scro-tum)

Gamete (gam-eet)

**Although puberty (adolescence) may begin as early as nine years of age, this subject matter is presented to aid in learning of body systems and diseases that affect these parts in various stages of the aging process.

URTICARIA
Ur-ti-car-i-a

Urticaria (hives) is a disorder of the integumentary and immune system.

It is a skin condition from a hypersensitive allergen. There is an allergic reaction to a normally harmless substance, such as plants, animals, drug medications, bug bites, food, or other material that can result in lesions (skin damage away from normal) on the arms and legs.

Signs and symptoms include itching, also known as pruritis. Scratching can lead to a larger size and spread of the white patches. Wheals are the raised lesions or patches that appear over the body.

*HINT TO SAY WORDS:

Urticaria (ER-tih-care-ee-uh)

Hypersensitive allergen (HY-pur-sen-sih-TIV AL-UR-GEN)

Wheal (WEEL)

Pruritis (PROO-eye-tis)

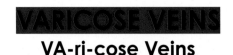

VARICOSE VEINS

VA-ri-cose Veins

Varicose veins are one of the diseases of **venous circulation** and affected by the **cardiovascular system**.

The veins are blood vessels that carry blood back to the heart. The **lower extremities** (legs) are affected by this health condition. Toward the surface of the skin of the legs, there are veins called the **saphenous** (superficial) veins. Deeper veins within the skin layer are responsible for carrying blood back to the heart. Blood in varicose veins collects in one area and blood flow slows, affecting circulation, and the valves in veins that open and close to keep blood flowing in one direction, no longer work well. **Blood pressure in legs increase** and **veins enlarge**.

Signs and symptoms include pain and swelling.

*HINT TO SAY WORDS:

Venous (VEE-nus)

Cardiovascular (CAR-dee-O-vas-cu-lar)

Saphenous (suh-FEE-nus)

WHOOPING COUGH
Whoo-ping Cough

Whooping cough is an infectious disease caused by the bacterium *Bordetella pertussis* of the respiratory system and activated by the immune system.

Pathogens are microorganisms (small organisms) including viruses, bacteria, fungi, and parasites that cause disease. Similar to coronavirus disease, whooping cough is transmitted or spread by person-to-person contact with respiratory droplets and is highly contagious.

Signs and symptoms of this infection include runny nose, sneezing, coughing, fever, inflammation of the larynx (voice box), trachea (TRAY-KEE-uh) (windpipe), and bronchi (tubes of lungs for air to pass through). Vaccines (substances used to make antibodies to provide immunity) are used to protect against whooping cough.

*HINT TO SAY WORDS:

Bordetella pertussis (bor-deh-tell-a per-tuh-sis)
Contagious (cun-tay-jus)

XERODERMA
Xe-ro-der-ma

Xeroderma is a skin disease affecting the integumentary system. It is characterized by excessively dry skin. There are many causes that can include aging, weather variations, dehydration (lack or not enough water) a vitamin A nutrition deficiency.

Xeroderma pigmentosum is a genetic disease of the skin and it is caused by ultraviolet light. Signs and symptoms can include severe sunburn when exposed to the sun and freckles on the skin, nervous system effects such as poor coordination and loss of hearing of the special senses.

*HINT TO SAY WORDS:

Xeroderma (Z-RO-der-ma)

Xeroderma pigmentosum (pig-men-TOE-sum)

Vitamin (VY-tuh-min)

Nutrition deficiency (NEW-trih-shun dee-fih-she-en-cee)

Genetic (geh-NET-ic)

YERSINIA PESTIS

Yer-si-ni-a Pes-tis

Yersinia pestis is bacteria which cause the infectious disease known as the plague. Microorganisms cause disease by invading the body and activating the immune system to release white blood cells and the inflammatory response to stay healthy. However, some diseases can be too much for the immune system to handle and prevent the body from protecting itself.

One of the historical pandemics was The Black Death of Europe, killing millions of people by *Yersinia pestis* which was spread to humans through fleas.

Presently, coronavirus disease 2019 (COVID-19) led to the pandemic caused by the SARS-CoV$_2$ spread by human to human transmission through respiratory droplets.

*HINT TO SAY WORDS:

Yersinia pestis (Yer-SIN-EE-uh).

Bacteria (bak-teer-ree-uh)

Plague (PLAYg)

Infectious (in-FEC-shus)

ZIKA VIRUS DISEASE
Zi-ka Vi-rus Dis-ease

Zika virus disease is an infectious disease activated by the lymphatic system and caused by the Aedes aegypti (EE-DEES EE-JIP-TY) mosquito. A mosquito becomes infected by biting an infected person who has Zika Virus. Once infected, the mosquito can pass the infected blood to another human through a bite. This is an example of how disease can be spread from insect to person to insect. Person-to-person contact is another way of transmitting this disease—during pregnancy when the mother passes it to the fetus and during sex between partners.

Signs and symptoms include asymptomatic, fever, headache, rash, muscle and joint pain, conjunctivitis (redness of the eye), and fatigue.

*HINT TO SAY WORD:

Zika (Z-kuh)

Transmission (TRANS-miss-shun)

Conjunctivitis (cohn-JUNK-tiv-eye-tiss)

**Although puberty (adolescence) may begin as early as nine years of age, this subject matter is presented to aid in learning of body systems and diseases that affect these parts in various stages of the aging process.

Wow! You have made it to the end of this book. Now, you have learned SOME of the many diseases that exist in the world. Some of these diseases may be a part of your family history, meaning that someone in your family has had these diseases or may be battling with them now—one or more of these illnesses. You may have been sick before, you might be sick now, or you know someone who is sick now, or has been sick before.

It is great to be educated on disease and health, as well as how the body is made and how all the parts work. However, it is even more important to focus on wellness, being happy and enjoying the life you were given—not just focused on disease (what went wrong in the body and all of the problems it can cause). You must believe that your life has meaning and purpose. You must know that you were put in this world for a special reason and believe that you CAN enjoy your life and be healthy.

This book must also serve as motivation and inspiration to you. It should give you hope. You should be able to learn about your body to be able to use what you have learned to improve your life. Every day when you open your eyes, you must know that you are HERE in this world. There is something special that you must do. You are here to have the things that you want. There is so much that you can do, and nothing can stop you.

At the end of this book, you will be provided with positive affirmations that you can say every day, any time of day. You must think positively. You must know that good things can happen to you and for you. Even as a child or teen, you can do special things. To have these special things, to do great things in the world, and to be all you can be, you must think it is possible. Things will happen in your life, no matter if you are young or old. You are a human being and you will have things happen to you and your family. Some of these things may be hard to handle and other things may be wonderful and good. No matter what you go through as you get older, it is important to think good thoughts. You must expect good things to happen for you and your family—no matter what it looks or seems like! You must think and say good things to feel good. As you feel good about life, family, and health, good things can happen for you.

These daily positive affirmations are presented in this book to help you focus on good things that you can think and say about yourself. You can use these words how you want to and for who you want. You can say them by yourself, or with a friend or family member. As you have already learned, your body is made of energy. All of the parts work together. Your body responds to your environment (what you are around, what you see, hear, eat, and the people you spend your time with). No one can stop you from thinking good things, saying good words, doing good in life, and having the best life you can. What you believe has nothing to do with anyone but you. You are here to live your best life, so live it! When things seem to go differently than you thought they should, just keep thinking, saying, and doing good.

DAILY Positive Affirmations for Health
I AM LOVED

I AM GOOD

I AM MADE SPECIAL

I AM HEALTHY

I AM STRONG

I AM HEALED

I AM FOCUSED

I AM POWERFUL

I AM LIMITLESS

I AM WHOLE

DAILY POSITIVE AFFIRMATIONS
FOR HEALTH CONTINUED...

I HAVE HEALTHY ATOMS WORKING IN MY BODY

I HAVE HEALTHY MOLECULES WORKING IN MY BODY

I HAVE HEALTHY CELLS WORKING IN MY BODY

I HAVE HEALTHY TISSUES WORKING IN MY BODY

I HAVE HEALTHY ORGANS WORKING IN MY BODY

I HAVE HEALTHY ORGAN SYSTEMS
WORKING IN MY BODY

ALL OF THE ATOMS, MOLECULES, CELLS, TISSUES, ORGANS, AND ORGAN SYSTEMS OF MY BODY ARE HEALTHY AND STRONG. I AM MADE OF GOOD ENERGY. I GIVE OFF GOOD ENERGY. GOOD ENERGY COMES BACK TO ME. I AM HAPPY AND REJOICE IN GOOD HEALTH AND HEALING EVERY DAY!

GLOSSARY

abdomen The middle part of the body between the chest and the pelvis that contains the organs of the digestive system.

alveoli Air sacs (cells) of the lungs that allow oxygen and carbon dioxide exchange.

antigens Foreign substances in the body that activate antibodies to be made by the immune system.

atom The smallest unit of an element that keeps its properties.

axon Part of the motor nerve cell that spreads from the spinal cord to a group of skeletal muscle fibers.

auditory Sense of hearing sound with the ears.

bile Substance made in the liver and stored in the gallbladder that mixes fat.

bilirubin Pigmented yellow bile made by the breakdown of old and worn red blood cells.

blood Connective tissue (fluid) in the body that carries oxygen and carbon dioxide, nutrients, removes waste products and carries disease-fighting white blood cells helps defend the body against disease.

brain Part of the nervous system and its activities that controls intelligence and sensation.

bronchus The tubes that allow the flow of air from the trachea and branches off to enter the lungs. When you inhale and exhale air passes to and from the lungs.

calcium Most abundant metal chemical element.

capillaries The smallest blood vessels in the body where oxygen and carbon dioxide exchange occurs.

carbon A nonmetal chemical element that bonds with other elements forming compounds.

cardiovascular system Body system that includes arteries, capillaries, heart, and veins for the circulation of blood through the body.

cell membrane Provides protection to the cell, holds organelles and other contents in the cell, while allowing nutrients and other substances to enter and waste products to exit.

central nervous system (CNS) Part of the nervous system that consists of the brain and spinal cord.

chlorine A chemical element and a gas.

cholesterol Lipid or fatty substance in the human cell membrane.

chromosome Molecule of deoxyribonucleic acid (DNA) in the human cell that contains a total of 46 separated into 23 pairs, one from each parent.

circulation Movement of fluid and the substances in it through the body.

colon The longest part of four parts of the large intestine.

conjunctiva Part of the eye that covers the inside of the eyelids and front of the eye. It makes clear water mucus.

contagious When a disease caused by pathogens that can spread from person to person.

cytoplasm Gel substance that holds all organelles and their parts in the cell, but not the nucleus.

dendrite Nerve cell process that carries a nerve impulse to cell body.

deoxyribonucleic acid (DNA) Blueprint for making new proteins in the cell. Molecule carrying gene instruction for growth, development, and how an organism works.

diabetes mellitus (DM) A condition characterized by too little production or making of insulin and results with too much glucose in the blood.

digestive system Directs the process of the chemical break down of food into nutrients to be used by the body.

diploid Complete set of 46 chromosomes from both male and female reproductive cells (mature sex cells are sperm and egg cells that contain one full set of chromosomes).

electrolytes Chemicals found in plasma of blood and have a positive and negative charge and conduct electricity in a solution. Sodium, potassium, calcium, magnesium, and bicarbonate (HCO_3^-) are electrolytes.

element A substance that cannot be divided anymore without losing its properties.

endocrine system Body system that includes parts: adrenal glands, ovaries, pancreas, parathyroid gland, pineal gland, pituitary gland, testes, thymus, and thyroid gland. This system makes and releases hormones in the bloodstream for the control of other body organs.

endoplasmic reticulum Organelle of network channels (web system) through the cytoplasm for the transport, support, storing, and putting together of molecules.

enzyme Protein molecule that speeds up the rate of chemical reactions in the body. It is necessary for the build-up and breakdown of substances.

epidemiology (ep-ih-DEE-ME-o-LO-GEE) The study of the science of understanding the cause, spread, prevention, and control of disease, health events, injury, and death among groups of people.

esophagus Digestive system organ that moves broken down food from the throat to the stomach.

estrogen Female sex hormone.

fetus An unborn offspring that develops from an embryo.

gametes Mature haploid male or female germ cell that must join to form a zygote

gene Located in chromosomes; it is a unit of heredity that plays a role in the making of one protein. A special sequence (arrangement, order) of DNA or ribonucleic acid (RNA) that codes for a molecule that has a job to do.

glucagon Hormone of the pancreas that increases production of glucose and triggers the liver to change glycogen into glucose.

glucose Sugar molecule found in food and in the blood of the human body.

glycogen Large sugar molecule or chains of glucose stored in the liver and skeletal muscle.

Golgi apparatus Organelle in the cytoplasm that processes proteins and lipids to the cell plasma membrane and other parts of cell organelles.

gustation Sense of taste.

haploid Single set of 23 chromosomes, *not paired* with one from female and male.

heart Muscular organ in the cardiovascular system that allows blood to be pumped through the blood vessels to carry oxygen and other important substances through the body.

hormone Chemical messenger made by endocrine glands in the human body.

hydrogen Most abundant nonmetal chemical gas element that forms water and other compounds.

immunity The body's ability to resist or fight against disease.

immunoglobulins (Ig) Antibodies. Examples are IgG, IgA, IgM, IgE, and IgD.

infectious disease Sickness that is caused by a pathogen (virus, bacterium, fungus, or parasite).

inflammation Chemical response by the body as result of infection, damage to the body, extreme heat, and chemicals.

integumentary system The system of the hair, skin, and nails and their parts.

kidney Urinary system organ that filters blood, makes urine, balances chemicals, and controls fluids in the body.

large intestine Organ allowing absorption of nutrients from the small intestine to the anus where waste is removed from the body.

lipids Fats in the human body.

liver Largest organ inside of the body and removes toxins from the blood, helps regulate blood sugar, and helps break down food, and many other things.

lymphatic vessels Connective tissue that carries lymph fluid and its components through the body.

lymph nodes lymph tissue that filter and destroy harmful substances and toxic cells that invade the body.

lysosome An organelle that contains digestive enzymes.

lungs Pair of organs of the respiratory system that allow oxygen to pass into the blood and remove the toxic gas carbon dioxide.

macrophage Important cells that are ready to meet an invading harmful pathogen, eat it, and take it to the white blood cell to make antibodies to fight against it to keep the body healthy later on if it comes into contact with it again.

magnesium A chemical element and mineral of the body.

menstrual cycle Female reproductive cycle for shedding of the lining of the uterus that occurs around every 28 days.

metabolism Process in the body that takes food and turns it into energy to be used by the body. All the processes in the body that include the buildup and breakdown of substances.

microorganism Small organism that can cause disease (bacteria, viruses, fungi, protozoa). Germ.

mitochondrion An organelle in the cell where energy is formed.

molecule Two or more atoms that come together to form a substance or compound.

motor neuron Nerve cell that creates a path from brain or spinal cord to muscle tissue or gland.

nerves Individual axons packaged together.

neuron A nerve cell.

nervous system The brain, spinal cord, and all nerve cells and their parts responsible for receiving and sending messages that tell the body what to do and how to do it. Emotions and how you feel about things are a part of this system.

nucleus The control center of the brain or cell within the human body.

nutrients Chemical substances found in food and available in the human body that allow growth and development.

olfaction Sense of smell.

onychomycosis Nail fungus or infection of the nail bed of the fingernails or toenails

organelle Small part of the cytoplasm of the cell that has its own special job to do in the human cell body.

ovum Mature female reproductive cell. When joined with a male reproductive cell, it forms an embryo.

oxygen Highly reactive nonmetal chemical element that combines with other elements forming compounds.

pancreas Organ belonging to both the endocrine and digestive system. Its job is to produce enzymes of the digestive system and produce hormones (insulin and glucagon) of the endocrine system.

pelvic Area of the body below the abdomen that contains organs of the urinary system and the male and female reproductive system.

pharynx Throat. Organ that allows both food and air to pass.

phospholipid Important fatty and phosphorus part that makes up the cell membrane.

phosphorous A nonmetal chemical element in the body.

plasma A clear fluid part of the blood the carries blood cells and many other materials that include clotting factors, proteins, electrolytes, glucose, hormones, minerals, bilirubin, urea, and creatinine.

potassium A chemical reactive element.

reproduction Produce offspring by the sex process.

Ribonucleic acid (RNA) A nucleic acid carrying instructions from DNA for the control of the protein-making process.

ribosome Organelle in the cytoplasm that is located on the endoplasmic reticulum of the cell.

sensory neuron Nerve cell of the nervous system that receives input.

sign In the presence of disease, an observation (what the doctor or examiner sees) and measurements (range) can be made to determine characteristics of illness.

small intestine Part of the intestine that has three parts and begins at the end of the stomach to the large intestine.

spleen Lymph organ that destroys old red blood cells and stores whole blood, contains white blood cells, and breaks down hemoglobin into heme and globin.

sodium A chemical reactive element.

stomach Digestive system organ that connects the esophagus to the small intestine. Allows food to mix with acid to break it down to be moved through the body into the blood to be used as energy.

symptom Something personal that the patient must tell you about his or her illness that the doctor cannot see or know without asking (an experience or feeling).

testes Glands in the scrotum of the male reproductive system that make and release the hormone testosterone.

testosterone Male sex hormone.

thymus gland Lymph organ of the endocrine system that triggers hormones to cause growth and development of white blood cells.

tongue Muscular organ of the digestive system that contains nerve cells to allow sense of taste and helps with talking and eating.

tonsils Lymph tissue that kills germs in the throat. Antibodies are made here.

triglycerides Main part of fat and oils in the human body that is formed from mostly hydrogen and carbon atoms.

uterus Part of the female reproductive system and special place of the body where the baby grows and develops.

vagina Area of the body that allows the baby to pass through into the outside world and allows readiness for human life to take place.

vitamin A chemical made and required by the body to maintain normal cell function. It can be found in foods to help support cell activity in the human body.

water A chemical element that is the main part of fluids of all living organisms. It is clear, tasteless, colorless, and does not contain carbon (inorganic).

zygote Diploid cell from the joining of two haploid gametes. A fertilized ovum.

CORONAVIRUS DISEASE (COVID-19): A LITTLE SIDE NOTE

At the time of this publication, our nation and the world is experiencing a global pandemic of this disease. There is so much to learn about this new infectious disease. In an effort to help others, many resources have been offered to assist with the understanding of this disease, although all is not factual. Here, I will present a few simple facts about COVID-19.

You can find reliable sources of information at:

www.CDC.gov

www.WHO.int

- Maintain a safe distance of 3 to 6 feet indoors and outdoors, avoid crowds and poorly ventilated indoor spaces, *and* wear a mask, which *may* provide protection against infected persons and respiratory droplets and large particles in the air
- Persons exposed to a person with suspected or confirmed COVID-19 should be quarantined for 14 days
- A person can be infected with this disease with or without symptoms
- A person can be infected before symptoms or during the incubation period of 4 to 5 days of exposure and onset of symptoms from 2-14 days
- A close contact is any person within 6 feet of an infected person for 15 minutes or more within 24-hour period
- A laboratory confirmed positive/negative test can present inaccurate results if taken too early after exposure or problems with how a lab performed test
- It is possible that a person who has had COVID-19, and recovered, can still become infected again and should be quarantined and retested
- There is a diagnostic test and an antibody test
- Diagnostic tests include molecular (polymerase chain reaction or PCR and detects viral load)

and antigen (rapid response detects proteins on surface of coronavirus).

- A negative test result means *at the time of the test*, you were likely not infected with COVID-19
- Antibody test determines if you had COVID-19 even if you did not have symptoms, and tests the antibodies in the blood or serum (clear part of blood after cell parts and clotting proteins are removed)
- Recovered adults do have a degree of immunity at least 90 days following COVID-19 infection
- Survivors of this disease have shown to produce antibodies that provide protection for months but there is still not enough information to suggest how long and the ability to protect against reinfection
- Young children under the age of 12 are still not eligible to be vaccinated and may become sick if exposed to a person with COVID-19
- Recommendations for testing *every two weeks* for people in contact with those outside of their household and unable to socially distance, and any travel outside the U.S.
- Vaccine is offered to provide protection for those 12 years of age and older
- NO VACCINE is 100% effective

- Authorized vaccines: BioNTech, Pfizer and Moderna (two doses, one month apart) and Janssen by Johnson and Johnson (one dose)
- Fully vaccinated status includes two weeks after second dose (Pfizer and Moderna) and two weeks after J & J's Janssen vaccine
- After exposure to a person or potential case of COVID-19, a *fully vaccinated* person should be tested within 3 to 5 days, whether symptoms are present or not
- No symptoms *does not* mean *no* COVID-19
- At this time, some individuals who have been fully vaccinated still became reinfected with COVID-19
- Virus infects a person and makes copies of its RNA. The more it copies, the more likely errors occur, causing mutations or variants.
- Variants: Alpha (detected in U.K., in U.S. 12/2020), Beta (South Africa 12/2020, in U.S. 1/2021), Gamma (detected in Brazil, U.S. 1/2021), Delta (India 12/2020, in the U.S. 3/2021), and Lambda (Peru 12/2020, in the U.S. 8/2021)
- Delta variant is a newly mutated (changed) version of the original strain

- Vaccines (approved through emergency authorization) may offer *some protection* against most variants
- Booster shot (third dose) or supplemental vaccine *may* be confirmed in the future, but currently *not* confirmed by demonstrated science and current health guidance
- Some geographical locations worldwide are now offering a third dose of Pfizer vaccine to at-risk adults ages 60 and older
- Pfizer is seeking emergency use authorization by the FDA for use of third dose (recommended after vaccination more than six months and within 12 months after vaccination)

COVID-19 IS NEW AND SCIENTISTS ARE STILL LEARNING ABOUT IT. INFORMATION IS UPDATED AS AVAILABLE BY PUBLIC HEALTH AUTHORITIES. Do all *you* can to protect *yourself* and *your* loved ones.

PUBLICATIONS

Cole, LaKeisha J., Rohrer, James E., and Schulze, Frederick W. (2011). "Academic worry and frequent mental distress among online doctoral students." *ProQuest/UMI Publishing.*

Rohrer, James E., Cole, LaKeisha J., and Schulze, Frederick W. (2012). "Cigarettes and self-rated health among online university students." *Journal of Immigrant and Minority Health, 14(3), 502-505.*

Other Books

From Failure to Success: Faith Changes the Outcome. 2019

HIIT Your Way to Fit. 2020

Child, You Are a Sower: Plant Seeds of Goodness. 2020

Learning About Nutrition: Just for Kids. 2020

Learning Letters with Animals: Just for Kids. 2020

Numbers and Shapes: Just for Kids. 2020

The Destiny Project: Journey to Becoming A Better You. 2020

L1M1TLE$$: Beating the Odds and Winning in Life. 2020

Website: www.thefaithoutcome.com

YouTube: True Wellness Consulting, LLC

Dr. LaKeisha J. Cole

Social Media:

Instagram: @drjeanco

TikTok: @drjeanco

Twitter: @DrLaKeishaJCol1

About
Dr. LaKeisha J. Cole

LaKeisha J. Cole, PhD, the author of *Faith Changes the Outcome; HIIT Your Way to Fit; The Destiny Project*; L1M1TLESS: Beating the Odds and Winning in Life; and a series of children's books, is an inspirational, motivational author and speaker on mind, body, and spiritual healing. She is passionate about helping people pursue the life they were destined to live through encouragement and guidance from the power within all of us. Knowing that life is a journey, and that there is growth and development for all, she desires to inspire others to be their best. This translates into understanding that there is a past, present, and future, and encouraging all to forgive the past, adjust as necessary to live a better present, and create the future desired.

Dr. Cole is an educator who holds educational degrees in public health epidemiology (doctorate), human nutrition (master's), and complementary and alternative medicine (bachelor's). She has taught in both graduate and undergraduate institutions of higher learning to assist students in their journeys to achieve their educational goals and dreams. She has also used her knowledge, skills, and abilities in her health and wellness consulting and other businesses to inspire and motivate people to live better, healthier, and more productive lives. Website: www.thefaithoutcome.com

Printed in the United States
by Baker & Taylor Publisher Services